If you are reading this book you are already on your way to making a positive change in your life. I recommend reading my first book, "Fitness Optimization," before reading this one. This isn't a marketing ploy; it's simply the best way to get you the most information- without being totally repetitive. These books are short, concise and relatively cheap, but I think you will find they are totally worthwhile if fitness is your goal.

I have been lucky enough to participate in sports my entire life. I realize many people do not have this opportunity, which is very unfortunate. I've always been good at creating my own personal workout plans, and one day it hit me. I want to be able to help people who haven't been as lucky as me, and teach them what they need to know in order to engineer their own fitness.

I will serve as your online personal trainer and at the end of this book I will provide my email address, that way if you have any questions you can contact me directly. I'm here to help you and I will do everything I can to assist you. I will provide detailed steps to leading a healthier and happier life, and also a detailed training schedule. This book is for anybody who wants to become healthy and fit but does not know where to start. Most of the literature on the subject of health and fitness is very intimidating and assumptive. But this book will start from scratch, construct a strong base of knowledge of the subject, and build from there. You've accepted that you need to make a change, now lets start acting on that decision. Forget about your current habits, past failures or anything else that is holding you back. This is a clean slate and it will be impossible for you to fail this time, just follow the steps.

I have been into fitness my entire life. I competed in flat water kayaking for years, trained in wrestling, boxing, jiu jitsu, swimming and running. Being healthy and fit is and always will be, at the very top of my priority list. It saddens me to see people who are unhappy with themselves and the person they have become. Let's get going!

Step 1:

Buy only healthy food! This may include salads (spinach, lettuce or kale), quinoa, tuna, lean chicken breast, whole wheat noodles, light pasta sauce, unsalted peanuts, fruit, coconut water, chia seeds, flax seeds (grind and refrigerate), whole wheat/ rye bread, natural nut butters, avocados, etc. There is a common myth that needs to be disregarded; this myth is that eating healthy must be extremely expensive. This is false because I have very little money, yet I am still able to eat way healthier than the average person. Yes McDonalds is cheap, but how much do you need to spend there to feel satisfied? When I used to eat there it would cost me at least $10, yet I can now eat a can of tuna ($1.50), a handful of peanuts, and part of a salad and feel satisfied. That's about $5 worth of food and it fills me up more because it has essential nutrients that my body needs, unlike McDonalds and other unhealthy foods. Eating out nowadays is expensive no matter where you go, so do yourself a favor and take the time to buy some decent groceries. I also can't believe how expensive microwave dinners have become. Most of these are horrible for you and contain very little food. I worked at a grocery store for six months and I was blown away by how much these expensive little things were –often bought by self-proclaimed 'broke' individuals. Never mistake convenience for nutrition.

By having only healthy foods and snacks at your disposal, you won't be able to cheat yourself and ruin your diet. As I mentioned in my first book, you are allowed to have a cheat day/ meal once a week, but I recommend going out for this cheat meal so that you don't pollute your living environment with tempting bad foods. Buy unhealthy foods only on the day that you wish to eat them, and make sure they are not around once you resume eating healthy.

Step 2:

Work on time management skills. You always have time for your own fitness and well being, so stop making excuses and start taking action. You need to determine at what point in the day you feel the most energized so that you can try to fit in exercise at that time. For me this optimal time is first thing in the morning or the early afternoon. I like to do my workouts early so that I don't have to worry about it for the rest of the day. I wasn't always like this; in the beginning I was too exhausted in the mornings to do anything. I soon realized that I wasn't sleeping enough and that I didn't have enough time or energy in the evening to workout either. This forced me to make the necessary change, which required sleeping more and working out in the morning or early afternoon. Experiment with different times, pick one that works for you and stick to it! Habits make everything exponentially easier.

Step 3:

The healthy eating aspect needs to start immediately, as far as the workouts go we need to start slow. Use light weight for every exercise to develop proper technique and range of motion. NEVER lift heavy by sacrificing technique and exercise quality. We want to ensure we are doing everything properly before we up the weight. I know you've probably heard this before but never lift with your back and always lift with your legs. I will describe proper technique for every exercise in the schedule that I provide. Lets get down to business.

The Schedule:

First I will provide some examples of nutritious meals and then I will get into the exact schedule. In the schedule I will put an asterisk (*) wherever I feel additional information needs to be provided. You will find these additional information sections at the end of every week in the exact order that they appear in the schedule.

Breakfast:

1) One serving of oatmeal with cranberries, a sliced banana, ground flaxseed, walnuts, cinnamon, almond milk and a tablespoon of maple syrup.

2) Half a cup of Quinoa with a tablespoon of brown sugar, sliced almonds, almond milk, chia seeds, ground flaxseed and an apple.

3) Large smoothie consisting of 1 banana, 4 dates, 1 tbs of natural peanut butter, 1 handful or kale/ spinach, 1 tbs of ground flaxseed, 1 tbs of chia seeds, 1 tbs of coconut oil, 1 teaspoon of honey, lots of cinnamon, 1 handful of assorted frozen fruit, unsweetened almond milk and coconut water (add until there's a sufficient amount of liquid in the smoothie.)

4) 2 eggs and two pieces of toast. On the toast I like to put natural peanut butter, a little bit of honey and cinnamon.

5) Egg banana pancakes. 1 banana blended up with two eggs. Make just like you would pancakes. I like to add cinnamon and a touch of maple syrup.

Lunch:

1) Burrito made with whole-wheat pita, avocado, black beans, quinoa/ brown rice, tomatoes, tuna, and sweet potato.

2) Kale & spinach salad. Add avocado, chickpeas, ground flaxseed and black beans. For dressing I like to use a tiny bit of balsamic vinegar.

3) Pan fried haddock and a sweet potato with coconut oil.

4) Tuna sandwich on rye or flaxseed bread. I like to add lettuce, tomato and a bit of siracha sauce or pesto.

5) Turkey wrap with hummus, goat cheese and spinach

Dinner

1) Spaghetti squash cooked in the oven. I like to add crushed tomatoes or a little bit of pesto.

2) Mango avocado salad. I use one mango and avocado, cut them up and add black beans, lettuce, jalapeños, quinoa, salsa and low fat corn chips. My personal favorite.

3) Mini pita pizzas. Add some pesto to pita bread with tomatoes, red pepper, onions and cheese. Bake the pita by the oven by itself first, add everything else and then put it back in the oven until the cheese melts

* More healthy dinners found in the bonus section at the end of the book

Some days will include two workouts, one in the morning (am) and one in the evening (pm). Keep in mind that Saturday is going to be a day of rest. It is not included in the schedule. I like to give a day of rest on Saturday and then a light workout on Sunday to prepare the muscles for the week ahead. As I mentioned in my first book "Fitness Optimization" stretching on your day off is a great idea, as it enforces the idea of muscle mobility. If you keep your muscles flexible you will better your range of motion, thus bettering your workout technique and reducing the risks of sustaining an injury. If you sustain a bad enough injury it can set you behind tremendously on your quest for fitness. Devise a personal stretching routine that works for you. You can Google search any muscle you want and you will find a suitable stretch for that particular muscle. Always remember to warm up properly before attacking a vigorous workout. In the first couple weeks of the schedule I will provide the warm ups in the workouts, after that it will be assumed that you have warmed up before beginning the workout. Here are some good dynamic warm-ups:

Warm-up A) 5- 10 minutes jump rope skipping, then 20 lunges

Warm-up B) 30 arm circles (15 each way), 5 burpees*, 20 squats*, 20 jumping jacks

Warm-up C) 2 X 30 reps* of: jumping jacks, high knees, seal jacks*

Warm-up D) 10 minute run (5 minutes out 5 minutes back)

*For a burpee, you start in the standing position, jump down until your chest is on the ground, do a pushup keeping your back flat, jump your legs up into a squatted position and spring yourself up into the air with your arms reaching to the sky. With practice this movement will become fluent, but it remains a very challenging exercise.

*Squats should be performed with your feet at shoulder width apart. Put your arms straight out in front of you and keep your back straight as you lower your bum to your ankles, keeping your legs parallel to one-another.

*I write sets as you see above. The first number is the number of sets and the second number is the number of repetitions per set. So if you see 4 x 20, that

means four sets of twenty reps per set. During a set you perform every exercise in order with no rest between exercise unless otherwise instructed.

*Seal jacks are like jumping jacks. Keep your arms straight but bring them together in front of your chest, instead of above your head.

At the end of every week there will be a short weekly review after the notes (where the asterisks are explained for the weekly schedule) section is complete. This will also discuss the following weeks schedule. Stick to this schedule and do not give up! If you feel like you have an average or higher than average fitness level, you can skip the first two weeks of the schedule. Lets get to work!

Don't forget that in order for this schedule to be a success in making you feel better, you must maintain a healthy diet. The diet is the most important part!

WEEK 1:

MONDAY- AM: 15 minute walk/ run.

- 3x10 reps of:

Pushups*, bodyweight squats, sit ups.

PM: Off

TUESDAY- AM: Off

PM: 5 minutes of skipping, 1 minute rest, 2 minutes of skipping*

WEDNESDAY- AM: 20 minute walk/jog

PM: Push ups: 20 reps, 1 min rest, 15 reps 45 seconds rest, 10 reps, 30 seconds rest. Repeat twice!

THURSDAY- AM: 8 minutes of skipping.

- 4 x 5 reps of 1 situp, 1 push up, 1 1 burpee

PM: 20 minute walk/jog

FRIDAY- AM: 6 minutes of as many sets as you can do. 10 squats, 5 pushups, 3 super burpees*.

PM: Off

SUNDAY- AM: 30 minute walk/ jog

PM: Off

NOTES

*Keep your arms at shoulder width apart, keep your back straight and make sure your chest touches the ground and that your arms are straight on every repetition.

*Make sure the skipping rope is long enough for you, you can skip in a stationary position, or you can move around while skipping. Once you get good you can do some double unders (rope goes under you twice per jump) or fast skipping.

*From now on, whenever you see the words super burpee, I want you to think 1 sit-up, 1 pushup, 1 burpee. I have dubbed this the super burpee because it is a superb exercise. Try to make this as smooth of a movement as you can. Do one complete sit-up, roll over onto your stomach and do a push up and then go immediately into a burpee.

Weekly Review:

     Congratulations on completing the first week of the program. Now that you have made working out a habit, it will become much easier for you to stick with the schedule. Next week the intensity will remain low but you will have less time off.

WEEK 2:

MONDAY- AM: 10 minute walk/jog

- 5 x 30 seconds plank* rest 2 minutes between sets

PM: 4 sets of: 20 sit ups, 10 push ups, 15 squats (rest as necessary between sets)

TUESDAY- AM: 100 jumping jacks, 50 seal jacks, 10 push ups

PM: 30 minute walk/ jog then: 3 x 25 reps of leg ups (bring knees to chest while on a chin up bar), mountain climbers, sit ups, leg lifts

WEDNESDAY- AM: 10 minute skip (try to do some double unders)

- 4 x 30 Kettlebell/ dumbbell swings* (rest 1 minute between sets)

PM: 3 sets of 25 lunges, 30 squats, 10 burpees

THURSDAY- AM: Off

PM: 1500 m row* - 3 sets of: 5 strict pull ups, * 20 mountain climbers*, 30 jumping jacks, 15 legs lifts*

FRIDAY- AM: Fitness Test: complete as many sets as you can in 5 minutes of: 10 squats, 8 sit ups, 6 pushups, 3 burpees*

PM: Off

SUNDAY- AM: 20 minute walk/ jog (try to cover as much distance as possible)

PM: 4 sets of 1 minute burpees (do as many reps as possible in the one minute and rest for 2 minutes between sets).

NOTES

* Planks are when you hover above the ground on your elbows and toes. Keep your back straight and your hips off the ground, stay stiff and hold the position.

* You can use dumbbells instead of kettle bells; it's just a little harder to hold onto them. Remember to start light, grip the kettle bell with two hands, let it swing between your legs, then thrust your hips while keeping your back straight

to swing the kettle bell up to eye level. Arms should be slightly bent, feet at shoulder width apart.

* Most indoor rowing machines have a digital display on the front of them so you can easily track the distance that you've covered.

*Strict pull-ups are done straight up and down with your palms facing away from you. Do not swing or kip, you want to minimize the momentum and maximize the difficulty. I want you to only do strict pull-ups from now on. Get assistance if necessary
by utilizing a weighted assistance mechanism found on certain pull-up machines.

* Mountain climbers are great for your core. To perform, hover above the ground on your toes with your arms straight. One at a time, bring your knees towards your chest in an alternating motion. Every time both legs go in and out you have completed one repetition.

* For leg lifts you want to lie flat on your back with your legs completely straight, bring your legs up from the ground until they are at 90 degrees relative to your torso and then lower them until they hover above the ground. Place hands under your bum.

* We will do this workout multiple times so that you can gauge your progress. See how many sets you can complete in the prescribed time duration, no rest!

Weekly Review:

That was a tough week, great work. Remember if you want to be successful you cannot miss a workout, no excuses! Next week will be a split, the first half will consist of mostly long endurance workouts and the second half will consist of short intense workouts. Prepare yourself and use your off time to rest! Remember to cool down after workouts, especially intense ones. I recommend stretching and using a foam roller or having a hot bath to relax your muscles.

WEEK 3:

MONDAY- AM: 20 minute jog (you should have worked your way up to a jog at this point in the program).

PM:100 sit-ups, 50 push ups, 20 pull-ups, 30 squats J*, 80 mountains climbers, 30 burpees (break the reps up in whichever way you want, just get it all done!)

TUESDAY- AM: Off

PM: 3 x 15-20 reps of: Bench Press, Flat Bench Pull, Dumbbell Fly's, Lat Pull Down, Alternating Lunges. (All of the above exercise descriptions are readily available on the Internet).

WEDNESDAY- AM: Off

PM: 25 minute jog

THURSDAY- AM: 8 x 2 minutes running 1 minute walking (try to bring your pace up past a jog on the 2 minutes*)

PM: Kettle bells: 3 sets of 30 swings, 20 cleans*, 10 push presses*, 4 Turkish getups* (rest 1:30 between sets)

FRIDAY- AM: 6 sets of 1 minute rowing, 1 minute burpees (rest 30 seconds between sets).

PM: Off

SUNDAY- AM: 3 sets of 1 minute of each exercise: jumping jacks, mountain climbers, burpees, flexed arm hang,* reverse crunches*, squats (rest 3 minutes between sets).

PM: 4 sets of 2 minutes light skipping, 1 minute fast skipping. No rest.

NOTES

* Squat jumps are performed just like a regular squat but you jump into the air about 1 foot upon extension of the legs.

* Try to run hard for these 2-minute sets, at minimum you should be jogging.

* Cleans are when you swing the kettle bell between your legs and then up into the cradle or rack position with one hand.

* Push press is when you rack the kettle bell and then push it straight up overhead.

* For a Turkish getup you must lie flat on your back, push the kettle bell upwards and slowly begin to stand and then reverse the movements until you are on your back again. The kettle bell should be held straight up the entire time, you must keep your eyes on the bell.

* Flexed arm hang is when you hang onto a chin-up bar with your arms bent and your eyes level with the bar. Stay up as long as you can and if you lose your grip get right back up.

*Reverse crunches are performed by lying flat on your back with your hands on the ground beside you. Your legs should be bent with your feet on the ground and you simply bring your knees up towards your chest and then back down to perform one repetition.

Weekly Review:

That was definitely a challenging week; let's keep up the progress. Next week we will perform the same fitness test from week two so that we can monitor your progress. The only difference will be that the test duration will be ten minutes long instead of five. Hopefully you are able to do more than double your sets from week two in this ten-minute period. Other than the fitness test next week won't be super difficult.

WEEK 4:

MONDAY- AM: 30 minute jog, every 5 minutes perform 3 burpees and 15 squats (stop the time when you do these exercises then resume jogging).

PM: 1500m row or 300m swim

TUESDAY- AM: Fitness test: Complete as many sets as you can in 10 minutes of: 10 squats, 8 sit ups, 6 push ups, 3 burpees.

PM: Off

WEDNESDAY- AM: Rowing: - 3 x 500m hard 1:30 rest between sets.

 PM: 21, 15, 9* reps of pull-ups (or flexed arm hang, reps become seconds), leg lifts, burpees.

THURSDAY- AM: 20 minute total workouts time: Skip for 3 minutes then perform squat jumps* for 1 minute x 5 for a total of 20 minutes.

PM: 1 hour jog (jog for 8 mins, walk for 2 mins).

FRIDAY- AM: In no more than 35 minutes complete 2000m of rowing, 500 skipping rope jumps, 1000m of running, 50 push ups, 10 pull-ups.

PM: Off

SUNDAY- AM: 20 minute jog, 5 burpees every 5 minutes*

PM: 4 sets of 15 super burpees, 30 jumping jacks

NOTES

* So for this workout you're going do to 21 reps of each exercise, then 15 reps and finally 9 reps. Try to Increase the speed and intensity of the reps as the reps decrease.

* Drop the skipping rope and immediately transition into the squat jumps, no rest.

* Keep the timer running when you drop and do your burpees, then immediately continue running.

Weekly Review:

Hopefully the fitness test went well and you were able to complete double or more the amount of sets that you did for your first test. Next week will have more rest.

WEEK 5:

MONDAY- AM: 6 x 1 minute sprint, 1 minute walk (running)

PM: 3 x 500m rowing, 40 kettle bell swings (rest 2 minutes between sets).

TUESDAY- AM: 1km run, 50 pull ups, 100 push ups, 150 squats, 1km run. (break the reps up however you like but make sure you do the runs only at the start and at the end).

PM: 20 min jog

WEDNESDAY: AM: Off

PM: Off

THURSDAY: AM: 2 x 30 reps of each exercise (minus burpees), 3 minutes rest between sets: Kettle bell swings, Russian twists*, push ups, kettle bell cleans, kettle bell squats, kettle bell curls, **15 burpees**.

PM: Off

FRIDAY: 50 double under skips (DU), 50 leg lifts, 40 DU, 40 push ups, 30 DU, 30 kettle bell swings, 20 DU, 20 mountain climbers, 10 DU, 10 Turkish getups, 5 DU, 5 burpee pull ups*

PM: 45 minute jog (Make this jog light, but keep a consistent pace).

SUNDAY- AM: 10-minute row, 10-minute skip.

PM: 3 X 25 reps of: Leg ins*, pikes*, Russian twists, flutter kicks*, reverse crunches. (At the end of every set do 1:30 plank and 6 Turkish getups with a kettle bell. Rest 2 minutes between sets).

NOTES

* For a Russian twist, sit down, lean back and let your legs hover above the ground. Rotate your core around side to side with your hands in front of you and your chest up. Let your hands touch the ground on either side of you to complete one full rep.

* Burpee pull-ups are just like regular burpees, except for that when you jump up you need to grab a bar and do a pull-up at the end to complete a full rep.

* Leg ins are done from the plank position. Once in position, bring your right knee to your right elbow, and then back. Do the same with your left side and that equates to two reps.

* Pikes are also done from the plank position. Simply arch your back and stick your bum into the air, returning to the plank position.

* For flutter kicks you must lie on your back. Hover your legs above the ground and move them up and down as if you were kicking in the water. Up and down on each legs is one repetition.

Weekly Review:

After 2 full days of rest you should be feeling good for some of the tough workouts to come next week. Make sure you're sticking to the exact schedule so that you can achieve maximum results. Next week has lots of run/ swim workouts and if you are able, you should try to do an equal amount of running and swimming. Take a moment and reflect upon how much your fitness level has increased since Week 1. Look at the type of workouts you are now able to conquer!

WEEK 6

MONDAY- AM: Swim laps or run for 30 minutes.

PM: 3 x 10-15 reps of:

Bench Press, Flat Bench Pull, Dumbbell Fly's, Lat Pull Down, Alternating Lunges, 1 minute flexed arm hang*

TUESDAY- AM: 2 x 1 minute on, 1 minute off, 30 seconds on of each exercise: burpees, jumping jacks, push ups, plank, squat jumps, reverse crunches, kettle bell swings, seal jacks (rest 2 minutes between sets).

PM: 20 min swim or run

WEDNESDAY- AM: Off

PM: If possible, measure 3 kilometers either with your car or a GPS watch. Time yourself doing this run. < 15 mins is awesome. < 18 mins is great. < 21 mins is good. < 24 mins is pretty good*

THURSDAY- AM: Off

PM: 4000-meter row

FRIDAY- AM: 35 minute total run, 4 mins jog, 1 min sprint x 7

PM: 6 Turkish getups, 30 swings, 30 cleans, 30 lunges, 20 upright rows, 30 squats.

SUNDAY- AM: Swim for 20 minutes straight (non-stop) or do a 30 minute jog.

PM: Off

NOTES

* 3 sets of 1 minute flexed arm hang

* Two sets total. One set means you have done every exercise for 1 min on, 1 min off, 30 seconds on. Don't rest between exercises, only between sets!

*This run is a fitness test and it will be done again before the program is complete.

Weekly Review:

Next week will be the second last week in the training program. During the final 8th week of the program we will repeat the two fitness tests that we have already done, so that you can revel in your progress. You will get adequate rest during this next week so that you will feel 100% for the final week of testing.

WEEK 7:

MONDAY- AM: For 15 minutes, every thirty seconds complete: 1 pull-up, 1 push up, 1 squat, 1 situp, 1 burpee (use the leftover time in the 30 seconds for rest).

PM: 3km run @ 70% of your fastest pace.

TUESDAY- AM: 1 x 1:00 on, 1:00 off, 1:00 on of each exercise: squat jumps, plank, burpees, flutter kicks, kettle bell swings.

PM: 15 minute jog

WEDNESDAY- AM: 15 x 1 minute hard running, 1 minute rest between sets.

PM: 3 sets of: 50 double under skips, 200m row, 30 reverse crunches, 20 push ups, 5 pull-ups, 30 squats.

THURSDAY- AM: Off

PM: 4 X 10-12 reps of: Bench Press, Flat Bench Pull, Dumbbell Fly's, Lat Pull Down, Alternating Lunges.

FRIDAY- AM: 5 sets of 6 burpee pull-ups (rest 1 min between sets).

PM: 3 x 500m rowing, 40 kettle bell swings (rest 2 minutes between sets).

SUNDAY- AM: 45 minute jog

PM: Off

NOTES

Weekly Review:

　　　You're almost there! Only one more week until the training program is complete. With all of this training there is almost no question that you will excel in the fitness tests next week!

WEEK 8:

MONDAY- AM: 10 pull ups, 20 burpees, 30 pushups, 40 sit ups, 50 squats

PM: 3 x 10-12 reps of: Bench press, Bench pull, Dumbbell fly's, Lat pull.

TUESDAY- AM: Aim to complete as many swimming laps as possible in 30 minutes.

PM: Jog 10 minutes out and run hard back.

WEDNESDAY- AM: Fitness test: Complete as many sets as you can in 10 minutes of: 10 squats, 8 sit ups, 6 push ups, 3 burpees.

PM: 20 minute jog

THURSDAY- AM: Off

PM: 25 minute light jog

FRIDAY- AM: 3 km timed run fitness test: < 15 mins is awesome. < 18 mins is great. < 21 mins is good. < 24 mins is pretty good.

PM: Off

SUNDAY- AM: Off

PM: Bonus fitness test: see how many burpees you can complete in 5 minutes! 50 reps is good. 70 reps is great. 85 reps is awesome. Anything over 100 reps is amazing!

Program Review:

Hopefully you enjoyed this two-month fitness program. If you managed to complete the entire thing, congratulations! My hope is that you have noticed an extreme improvement in your fitness level, and that you feel like a healthier person. Hopefully this program has drastically expanded your knowledge of exercise, and given you the tools necessary to achieve your goals

Conclusion:

Now that the two-month program is complete, it is important that you keep fitness high on your priority list. This should be easy if you have followed the program, because working out and being healthy will have rapidly become a good habit. Do not let yourself become one of the statistics of people who have achieved a healthy lifestyle, and then quickly plummeted back into their unhealthy ways- often times ending up worse-off than they were before. You now have a good base of fitness knowledge, basic nutrition advice, simple warm up routines and a diverse workout schedule. Use this knowledge to manage your lifestyle. You can create a training schedule for yourself based on the one you just completed. It's easy to alter the workouts in any way that you please, making them easier, or more difficult depending on what you want, simply by altering the sets, repetitions, or overall durations. In addition, you could extend the 8-week program by repeating each weekly exercise plan (do week 1 workouts for two weeks, week 2 workouts for two weeks, etc.). Do this only if you feel as though your body needs more time to adapt and progress.

If you have any questions about any of the material found in this book, feel free to contact me by email at: **johnmayo@hotmail.com**
I will do my best to get back to you ASAP. This is my thanks for purchasing this book.

Bonus Material:

Here are some more great workouts that I enjoy completing on a regular basis:

1) 4 sets of 1 min exercise 30 seconds alt with 2 min rest between sets:
Kettle bell swings, alt = jumping jacks, kettle bell clean and press, alt = squats, pull-ups, alt = burpees, kettle bell curls, alt = reverse crunches.

2) 3 sets of:
400m run, 30 burpees, 50 double unders, 25 push ups, 20 squat jumps, 3 alternating kettle bell cleans, 30 lunges.

3) 4 x 25 reps of:

Reverse crunches, leg lifts, leg ins, Russian twists, U-sits, flutter kicks.

4) 1 hour run, every 4 minutes complete 5 burpees, 10 push ups, 15 squats.

5) Double unders/ burpee descending ladder: 10 burpees, 10 double unders, 9 burpees, 9 double unders, 8 burpees, 8 double unders.. all the way down to 1 and 1. (You can substitute anything in for double unders, squat jumps, jumping jacks, sit-ups).

<u>Here are some of my favorite alternative healthy food choices:</u>

1) Quinoa Chilli: 1/2 cup Quinoa, can of black beans, 1 large sweet potato, can of crushed tomatoes, 1 onion, 3 cloves garlic, salt and pepper, 2 tsp cumin, 2 tbl chilli powder. Optional: 2 cups vegetable broth, avocado, cilantro

2) Chili Lime Kale Chips: Preheat an oven to 350 degrees F (175 degrees C). Line a non-insulated cookie sheet with parchment paper. With a knife, carefully remove the leaves from the thick stems and tear into bite size pieces. Wash and thoroughly dry kale with a salad spinner. Drizzle kale with lime juice and sprinkle with chilli powder. Bake until the edges brown but are not burnt, about 10 to 15 minutes.

3) Greek Chickpea Salad: combine one can or two cups of soaked chickpeas, diced red bell pepper, diced yellow pepper, diced red onion, chopped fresh basil, diced cherry tomatoes, diced cucumber, feta cheese, diced olives. Add an olive oil based dressing with added balsamic, apple cider vinegar, lemon juice, pepper and sea salt.